DELICIOUSLY ALLERGY-FRIENDLY

A COOKBOOK FOR HEALTHY LIVING

shittu kolawole

TABLE OF CONTENT

INTRODUCTION

Welcome to "Deliciously Allergy-Friendly: A Cookbook for Healthy Living." This book is your guide to navigating the world of food allergies with confidence and creativity. Whether you or a loved one is newly diagnosed or have been managing food allergies for years, this cookbook is designed to help you enjoy delicious, safe, and nutritious meals.

Understanding the Challenge
Food allergies affect millions of people worldwide, impacting individuals of all ages. For those living with food allergies, everyday activities like grocery shopping, meal preparation, dining out, and attending social events can be fraught with challenges. The need to avoid specific allergens requires constant vigilance and can often feel overwhelming.

Despite these challenges, it is entirely possible to live a healthy and fulfilling life with food allergies. The key is education, preparation, and a positive approach to discovering new foods and recipes that fit within your dietary restrictions.

The Purpose of This Cookbook
This cookbook aims to:

Educate and Inform: Provide comprehensive information about food allergies, including common allergens, symptoms, diagnosis, and management strategies.
Empower and Equip: Offer practical advice on setting up an allergy-friendly kitchen, understanding food labels, and making safe ingredient substitutions.
Inspire and Delight: Present a wide variety of delicious recipes that are free from common allergens, proving that you don't have to sacrifice flavor or variety to eat safely.
Support and Connect: Offer guidance on navigating social situations, dining out, and traveling with food allergies, ensuring you can fully participate in life's activities.
What to Expect

In this book, you'll find:

Detailed Information on Food Allergies: Understand the science behind allergic reactions, the importance of proper diagnosis, and the latest in allergy management.

Practical Tips for an Allergy-Friendly Kitchen: Learn how to set up your kitchen, plan meals, shop for groceries, and read labels to avoid allergens.

Tasty and Safe Recipes: Enjoy a collection of recipes for breakfasts, lunches, dinners, snacks, and desserts that cater to various dietary restrictions without compromising on taste.

Strategies for Social and Emotional Well-Being: Discover how to handle the emotional and social aspects of living with food allergies, from managing anxiety to advocating for yourself in social situations.

Resources and Support: Access a list of valuable resources, including websites, books, support groups, and medical advice to help you on your journey.

A Note on Safety

While every effort has been made to ensure the recipes in this book are safe for those with food allergies, it is crucial to remain vigilant. Always double-check ingredient labels, be aware of potential cross-contamination, and consult with your healthcare provider if you have any concerns.

Embracing the Journey
Living with food allergies can be challenging, but it also presents an opportunity to explore new foods, develop creative cooking skills, and build a supportive community. This cookbook is here to help you embrace that journey, providing you with the tools and confidence to enjoy a healthy and delicious allergy-friendly lifestyle.

Thank you for choosing "Deliciously Allergy-Friendly: A Cookbook for Healthy Living." Let's embark on this culinary adventure together, turning food allergies from a limitation into an opportunity for discovery and delight

CHAPTER ONE

UNDERSTANDING FOOD ALLERGIES

Food allergies are immune reaction that occur after consuming certain foods. Even tiny amounts of these foods can trigger symptoms ranging from mild to severe.Here are some of the most common food allergens

Gluten

Found in wheat, barley, and rye, gluten can cause serious reactions in individuals with celiac disease or non-celiac gluten sensitivity. Symptoms may include digestive issues, skin rashes, and fatigue.

Dairy

Milk and other dairy products contain proteins like casein and whey that can trigger allergic reactions. Symptoms often include digestive problems, skin reactions, and respiratory issues.

Nuts

Tree nuts (such as almonds, walnuts, and cashews) and peanuts are common allergens. Reactions can range from mild hives to severe anaphylaxis.

Soy

Soybeans and soy products can cause allergic reactions, particularly in children. Symptoms may include digestive upset, skin reactions, and respiratory problems.

Eggs

Egg allergies are common in children but can also affect adults. Symptoms can include skin reactions, respiratory issues, and digestive problems.

Fish and Shellfish

Seafood allergies can cause severe reactions and are more common in adults. Symptoms may include digestive upset, skin reactions, and anaphylaxis.

Symptoms and Diagnosis

Symptoms of Food Allergies
Symptoms can vary widely and may include:

Skin reactions: Hives, itching, eczema
Gastrointestinal
Symptoms:Nausea,vomiting,diarrhoea,
abdominal pain

Respiratory symptoms: Nasal congestion,
wheezing, shortness of breath

Anaphylaxis
 A severe and potentially life-threatening
allergic reaction that demands immediate
medical attention. Symptoms of anaphylaxis
may include difficulty breathing, a drop in
blood pressure, and loss of consciousness.

diagnosis of food allergies

Diagnosing food allergies typically involves
several steps:

Medical History: Your doctor will discuss your symptoms and dietary habits in detail.

Elimination Diet: This involves removing suspected allergens from your diet and gradually reintroducing them to observe any reactions.

Skin Prick Test: Small amounts of potential allergens are introduced to your skin to observe any reactions.

Blood Test: This measures the immune system's response to specific foods by checking for allergy-related antibodies.

managing food allergies in daily life

Managing food allergies requires careful planning and vigilance. Here are some strategies to help you navigate daily life with food allergies:

Read Labels

Always check ingredient lists for potential allergens. Be aware that allergens can be listed under different names, so familiarise yourself with alternative names for common allergens.

Ask Questions

When dining out, inform the staff about your allergies and ask about ingredients and preparation methods. Don't hesitate to ask for detailed information to ensure your meal is safe.

Prepare Meals at Home

Cooking at home enables you to manage the ingredients and prevent cross-contamination.. Use separate utensils and cookware for allergen-free meals to prevent accidental exposure.

Carry Medication

Always have your prescribed medication, such as antihistamines or an epinephrine auto-injector, on hand. Ensure that those around you know how to administer the medication in case of an emergency.

Educate Others

Make sure family, friends, and caregivers are aware of your allergies and know how to respond in case of an emergency. Educating others can help create a safer environment for you.

Plan Ahead

When travelling or attending social events, plan ahead to ensure you have safe food options. Pack allergy-friendly snacks and meals if necessary, and communicate your needs to hosts or event organisers.

Understanding food allergies and how to manage them is crucial for maintaining your health and well-being. By being informed and prepared, you can enjoy a variety of delicious and safe meals without compromising your safety.

CHAPTER TWO

ALLERGY-FRIENDLY INGREDIENTS

In this chapter, we explore essential ingredients and substitutes that cater to various food allergies, ensuring you can still enjoy delicious and nutritious meals while managing your dietary restrictions.

Substitutes for Common Allergens

Gluten Substitutes
Gluten-Free Flours: Almond flour, coconut flour, rice flour, and gluten-free oat flour are versatile alternatives for baking and cooking.

Gluten-Free Grains: Quinoa, millet, buckwheat, and sorghum can be used as nutritious substitutes for wheat-based grains.

Dairy Alternatives

Plant-Based Milks: Almond milk, soy milk, coconut milk, and oat milk provide dairy-free options for beverages, cooking, and baking.

Non-Dairy Yoghourts: Made from coconut, almond, or soy, these yogurts offer creamy textures without dairy.

Nut Replacements
Seeds: Sunflower seeds, pumpkin seeds, and hemp seeds can be ground into flour or used as toppings for added crunch.

Seed Butters: Sunflower seed butter and pumpkin seed butter are nutritious alternatives to peanut butter.

Soy-Free Options
Coconut Aminos: A soy sauce alternative made from coconut sap, suitable for those avoiding soy.
Chickpea Flour: Used in cooking and baking as a soy-free alternative for thickening and binding.

Egg Replacements
Flaxseed or Chia Seed Eggs: Ground flaxseeds or chia seeds mixed with water can substitute eggs in baking recipes.

Tips for Reading Labels and Shopping

Navigating grocery aisles requires careful scrutiny of food labels to avoid allergens. Here's how to decode labels effectively:

Check Ingredient Lists: Look for common allergens such as wheat, dairy, nuts, soy, eggs, fish, and shellfish. Manufacturers must clearly label these allergens.

Understand Allergen Warnings: Statements like "Contains: [allergen]" or "May contain traces of [allergen]" indicate potential cross-contamination risks.

Look for Certification: Products labelled with certifications like "Gluten-Free," "Dairy-Free," or "Nut-Free" meet specific allergen-free standards.

Learn Alternative Names: Ingredients like casein (a milk derivative), albumin (found in egg whites), and legume (a term including peanuts and soybeans) might not be immediately recognizable.

Pantry Essentials for an Allergy-Friendly Kitchen

Stock your kitchen with these essential items to create allergy-friendly meals with ease:

Gluten-Free Flours: Almond flour, coconut flour, and gluten-free oats.

Dairy Alternatives: Plant-based milks, such as almond, soy, or oat milk.

Nut-Free Spreads: Sunflower seed butter or tahini.

Allergen-Free Oils: Olive oil, coconut oil, or avocado oil.

Alternative Sweeteners: Maple syrup, honey, or coconut sugar.

Herbs and Spices: Enhance flavor without allergens.

Safe Snacks: Fresh fruits, vegetables, and homemade trail mix.

Baking Essentials: Baking powder, baking soda, and gluten-free starches.

Safe Condiments: Mustard, vinegar, and allergy-friendly salad dressings.

By stocking your pantry with these ingredients and following tips for label reading, you can confidently create allergy-friendly dishes that are both delicious and safe. Whether you're preparing breakfast, lunch, dinner, or snacks, these substitutes and shopping strategies ensure you maintain a healthy and enjoyable culinary experience while managing food allergies.

CHAPTER 3

RECIPES

This chapter is the heart of your allergy-friendly journey. It features a variety of delicious, nutritious, and safe recipes tailored to accommodate common food allergies. Each section includes recipes for different meals and occasions, ensuring you can enjoy flavorful dishes without compromising on dietary restrictions.

Breakfast
1. Smoothies and Juices
Berry Blast Smoothie
Ingredients: 1 cup almond milk, 1 banana, 1 cup mixed berries, 1 tablespoon chia seeds, 1 tablespoon honey

Instructions: Blend all ingredients until smooth. Serve chilled.

Green Power Juice

Ingredients: 2 cups spinach, 1 cucumber, 2 green apples, 1 lemon, 1-inch ginger piece

Instructions: Juice all ingredients together. Stir and serve immediately.

2. Allergy-Friendly Pancakes

Gluten-Free Banana Pancakes

Ingredients: 1 cup gluten-free flour, 1 teaspoon baking powder, 1 mashed banana, 1 cup almond milk, 1 teaspoon vanilla extract

Instructions: Mix all ingredients in a bowl. Cook on a non-stick skillet over medium heat until bubbles appear. Flip and cook until golden brown. Serve with maple syrup.

3. Breakfast Bowls and Porridge

Quinoa Breakfast Bowl

Ingredients: 1 cup cooked quinoa, 1/2 cup almond milk, 1 tablespoon maple syrup, 1/2 teaspoon cinnamon, fresh berries

Instructions: Combine quinoa, almond milk, maple syrup, and cinnamon in a bowl. Top with fresh berries.

Lunch
1. Salads and Dressings

Mediterranean Chickpea Salad
Ingredients: 1 can chickpeas (drained), 1 cucumber (diced), 1 bell pepper (diced), 1/4 cup red onion (chopped), 1/4 cup olive oil, 2 tablespoons lemon juice, salt and pepper to taste
Instructions: Mix chickpeas, cucumber, bell pepper, and red onion in a bowl. Drizzle with olive oil and lemon juice. Season with salt and pepper. Toss well and serve.

2. Soups and Stews
Butternut Squash Soup
Ingredients: 1 butternut squash (peeled and cubed), 1 onion (chopped), 2 garlic cloves (minced), 4 cups vegetable broth, 1 teaspoon ground cumin, salt and pepper to taste
Instructions: Sauté onion and garlic in a pot until softened. Add squash, broth, and cumin. Simmer until squash is tender. Blend until smooth. Season with salt and pepper.
3. Sandwiches and Wraps

Turkey and Avocado Wrap
Ingredients: 1 gluten-free wrap, 3 slices turkey breast, 1/2 avocado (sliced), 1 cup mixed greens, 1 tablespoon hummus
Instructions: Spread hummus on the wrap. Layer turkey, avocado, and greens. Roll firmly and cut in half.

Dinner

1. Main Courses

Lemon Herb Chicken
Ingredients: 4 chicken breasts, 1/4 cup olive oil, 2 lemons (juiced), 3 garlic cloves (minced), 1 tablespoon dried oregano, salt and pepper to taste
Instructions: Marinate chicken in olive oil, lemon juice, garlic, oregano, salt, and pepper for 30 minutes. Grill or bake at 375°F until cooked through.

2. Sides and Vegetables

Roasted Brussels Sprouts
Ingredients: 1 pound Brussels sprouts (halved), 2 tablespoons olive oil, 1 teaspoon garlic powder, salt and pepper to taste

Instructions: Toss Brussels sprouts with olive oil, garlic powder, salt, and pepper. Roast at 400°F for 25-30 minutes until crispy.
3. Pasta and Grains

Quinoa and Veggie Stir-Fry
Ingredients: 1 cup cooked quinoa, 1 bell pepper (sliced), 1 zucchini (sliced), 1 cup broccoli florets, 2 tablespoons coconut aminos, 1 tablespoon olive oil
Instructions: Sauté vegetables in olive oil until tender. Add quinoa and coconut aminos. mix thoroughly and keep cooking for another five minutes.

Snacks
1. Energy Bars and Balls

No-Bake Energy Balls
Ingredients: 1 cup gluten-free oats, 1/2 cup sunflower seed butter, 1/4 cup honey, 1/4 cup flaxseeds, 1/4 cup dark chocolate chips
Instructions: Mix all ingredients in a bowl. Shape into balls and chill in the refrigerator for 1 hour before serving.

2. Crackers and Dips
Homemade Hummus
Ingredients: 1 can chickpeas (drained), 1/4 cup tahini, 2 tablespoons olive oil, 1 lemon (juiced), 2 garlic cloves, salt to taste
Directions: grind all ingredients in a food processor until it becomes smooth. Serve with veggie sticks.

3. Fruits and Veggies

Apple Nachos
Ingredients: 2 apples (sliced), 2 tablespoons sunflower seed butter, 1 tablespoon honey, 1 tablespoon mini chocolate chips
Instructions: Arrange apple slices on a plate. Drizzle with sunflower seed butter and honey. Sprinkle with chocolate chips.

Desserts
1. Cakes and Cookies

Chocolate Chip Cookies
Ingredients: 1 cup gluten-free flour, 1/2 teaspoon baking soda, 1/2 teaspoon salt, 1/2 cup coconut oil, 1/2 cup coconut sugar, 1 egg

substitute, 1 teaspoon vanilla extract, 1 cup dark chocolate chips

Instructions: Combine dry ingredients in one bowl and wet ingredients in another.. Combine both and fold in chocolate chips. Scoop onto a baking sheet and bake at 350°F for 10-12 minutes.

2. Pies and Tarts

Berry Tart

Ingredients: 1 gluten-free pie crust, 2 cups mixed berries, 1/4 cup honey, 1 tablespoon lemon juice

Instructions: Mix berries, honey, and lemon juice. Pour into pie crust and bake at 375°F for 30-35 minutes.

3. Ice Cream and Frozen Treats

Banana Ice Cream

Ingredients: 4 bananas (sliced and frozen), 1/4 cup almond milk, 1 teaspoon vanilla extract

Instructions: Blend frozen bananas, almond milk, and vanilla extract until smooth. Serve right away or freeze for a more solid texture.Each recipe in this chapter is crafted to be allergy-friendly, ensuring you can enjoy a wide variety of meals without compromising on taste or safety. Happy cooking!

CHAPTER 4

MEAL PLANNING AND PREPARATION

In Chapter 4 of "Deliciously Allergy-Friendly: A Cookbook for Healthy Living," we delve into effective strategies for meal planning and preparation that cater to individuals managing food allergies. This chapter focuses on optimizing your kitchen routines to ensure convenience, variety, and nutritional balance in your meals.

Weekly Meal Plans
Creating weekly meal plans helps streamline your cooking process and ensures you have allergy-friendly meals ready throughout the week. Here's how to create effective meal plans

Plan aroundallergen-frestaples: Incorporate allergy-friendly ingredients and substitutes into your meals to avoid common allergens.

Balance Nutrients: Ensure each meal plan includes a variety of nutrients and food groups to support overall health.

Consider Batch Cooking: Plan meals that can be easily doubled or tripled to save time and effort during busy days.

Rotate Recipes: Include a mix of familiar favorites and new recipes to keep meals exciting while accommodating dietary restrictions.

Batch Cooking Tips

Batch cooking allows you to prepare larger quantities of food in advance, making it easier to manage meals throughout the week. Here are some batch cooking tips:

Choose Versatile Recipes: Select recipes that can be easily adapted or transformed into different meals.

Use Freezer-Friendly Containers: Invest in freezer-safe containers to store pre-cooked meals and ingredients for future use.

Label and Date: Label containers with the contents and date of preparation to keep track of freshness.

Thaw Properly: Plan ahead to thaw frozen meals in the refrigerator overnight or use microwave-safe techniques for quick thawing.

Storing and Reheating Meals

Proper storage and reheating techniques are essential for maintaining food safety and quality:

Storage Containers: Use airtight containers to store leftovers and prepped ingredients in the refrigerator or freezer.

Reheating Safely: Reheat meals thoroughly to an internal temperature of at least 165°F (74°C) to ensure food safety.

Avoid Cross-Contamination: Use separate utensils and clean surfaces when handling allergen-free meals to prevent cross-contact. By implementing these meal planning and preparation strategies, individuals with food allergies can effectively manage their dietary needs while enjoying flavorful and nutritious meals. Whether preparing breakfasts, lunches, dinners, or snacks, Chapter 4 equips readers with practical tips to enhance their culinary routines and simplify their allergy-friendly lifestyles.

CHAPTER 5

SPECIAL OCCASION AND HOLIDAY

Special occasions and holidays are times of joy, celebration, and gathering with loved ones. However, for those managing food allergies, these events can also bring anxiety and challenges. Chapter 5 of "Deliciously Allergy-Friendly: A Cookbook for Healthy Living" provides practical advice and delicious recipes to ensure that you can safely enjoy festive occasions without compromising on fun or flavor.

Planning Ahead for Special Occasions

1. Communication is Key
Discuss Allergies Early: Inform hosts about your food allergies well in advance of the

event. This gives them time to plan and accommodate your needs.

Offer to Help: Volunteer to bring a dish or help with food preparation to ensure there are safe options available.

2. Create an Action Plan

Emergency Plan: Have an emergency action plan in place and make sure someone at the event is aware of it. Carry your emergency medication, such as antihistamines and an epinephrine auto-injector.

Safe Foods List: Prepare a list of safe foods and ingredients that can be shared with the host or used to verify dishes.

3. Bring Your Own Food

Personal Dish: Bring a dish that you know is safe for you to eat. This ensures that you have at least one allergen-free option and can enjoy the meal with everyone else.

Portable Snacks: Carry portable, allergen-free snacks in case safe options are limited.

Tips for Common Holiday Celebrations

Thanksgiving
Turkey and Trimmings: Check for hidden allergens in pre-seasoned or pre-stuffed turkeys. Consider preparing a simple, allergy-friendly roasted turkey

.

Stuffing: Use gluten-free bread or grain-based stuffing with safe herbs and spices.
Sides and Sauces: Make classic sides like mashed potatoes with dairy-free alternatives and ensure gravies are free of allergens.

2. Christmas and Hanukkah
Holiday Dinners: Plan allergy-friendly main courses and sides. Use safe ingredients to prepare traditional dishes.

Baking Traditions: Modify holiday cookie and dessert recipes with allergen-free substitutes.

Consider using gluten-free flour, dairy-free margarine, and egg replacers.

Latkes and Sufganiyot: For Hanukkah, prepare potato latkes with safe oil and flours, and make sufganiyot (jelly-filled donuts) with allergy-friendly ingredients.

3. Halloween

Safe Treats: Provide allergy-friendly treats for trick-or-treaters. Many companies offer safe alternatives that are clearly labeled.

Non-Food Options: Consider non-food treats like small toys, stickers, or glow sticks to include all children

.

4. Easter

Egg Hunts: Use plastic eggs filled with safe treats or non-food items. Be cautious with traditional chocolates and candies, checking labels for allergens

.

Brunch Ideas: Create a safe Easter brunch with dishes like dairy-free quiche, gluten-free pastries, and fresh fruit salads.

5. Birthdays and Parties

Customized Cakes: Bake or order allergen-free cakes or cupcakes. There are many recipes and bakeries that specialize in allergy-friendly desserts.

Party Foods: Serve a variety of allergen-free snacks and dishes, such as veggie platters, fruit trays, and safe chips with dips.

Recipes for Special Occasions

1. Allergy-Friendly Roast Turkey

Ingredients: Turkey, olive oil, fresh herbs, garlic, salt, pepper.

Instructions: Rub the turkey with olive oil and season with fresh herbs, garlic, salt, and pepper. put in the oven with an internal temperature of 165°F (74°C).

2. Gluten-Free Stuffing

Ingredients: Gluten-free bread, onions, celery, garlic, chicken broth, herbs (sage, thyme, rosemary).

Instructions: Sauté onions, celery, and garlic. Mix with cubed gluten-free bread, herbs, and chicken broth. Bake until golden brown.

3. Dairy-Free Mashed Potatoes
Ingredients: Potatoes, dairy-free butter, almond milk, salt, pepper.
Instructions: Boil and mash potatoes. Mix in dairy-free butter, almond milk, salt, and pepper until creamy.

4. Egg-Free Holiday Cookies
Ingredients: Gluten-free flour, dairy-free butter, sugar, egg replacer, vanilla extract.
Instructions: Cream together dairy-free butter and sugar. Add egg replacer and vanilla. Mix in gluten-free flour. Shape cookies and bake until golden.

5. Hanukkah Latkes
Ingredients: Potatoes, onion, gluten-free flour, egg replacer, salt, pepper, oil for frying.
Instructions: Grate potatoes and onion. Mix with gluten-free flour, egg replacer, salt, and pepper. Fry in hot oil until crispy.

6. Allergen-Free Birthday Cake
Ingredients: Gluten-free flour, dairy-free butter, sugar, egg replacer, vanilla extract, baking powder.
Instructions: Mix all ingredients and bake in a cake pan. Frost with dairy-free frosting once cooled.

Navigating Social Situations

1. Buffets and Potlucks
Bring Your Own Dish: Ensure there's at least one safe option by bringing your own allergen-free dish to share.
Avoid Cross-Contamination: Be cautious at buffets where serving utensils might transfer allergens between dishes.

2. Dining Out
Choose Wisely: Select restaurants known for accommodating food allergies. Call the restaurant ahead to discuss your dietary needs.

Communicate Clearly: Inform the waiter and chef about your allergies. Ask about ingredients and preparation methods.

3. Family Gatherings

Set Expectations: Talk to family members about your food allergies and discuss safe food options before the event.

Educate and Advocate: Use these gatherings as an opportunity to educate others about food allergies and safe cooking practices.

By planning ahead and using the strategies outlined in this chapter, you can confidently enjoy special occasions and holidays while managing food allergies. With delicious, allergen-free recipes and practical tips, you can create memorable celebrations that are both safe and enjoyable for everyone.

CHAPTER 6

KIDS' CORNER

In Chapter 6 of "Deliciously Allergy-Friendly: A Cookbook for Healthy Living," we focus on making mealtime enjoyable, safe, and nutritious for children with food allergies. This chapter provides fun and easy-to-follow recipes that cater to kids' tastes and dietary needs, along with tips for parents on managing allergies in children.

Fun and Nutritious Recipes for Kids

1. Breakfast
Rainbow Fruit Parfait
Ingredients: 1 cup coconut yogurt, 1 cup mixed berries, 1 banana (sliced), 1/2 cup granola (gluten-free)

Instructions: Layer coconut yogurt, berries, banana slices, and granola in a clear cup. Repeat layers and serve.

2. Lunch
Chicken Veggie Nuggets
Ingredients: 1 pound ground chicken, 1 cup finely chopped broccoli, 1 cup grated carrots, 1/2 cup gluten-free breadcrumbs, 1 egg substitute

Instructions: Combine all ingredients in a bowl. Shape into small nuggets and place on a baking sheet. Bake at 375°F for 20-25 minutes until golden brown.

Mini Pita Pizzas
Ingredients: Gluten-free pita bread, 1/2 cup tomato sauce, 1 cup dairy-free cheese, assorted toppings (pepperoni, olives, bell peppers)

Instructions: Spread tomato sauce on pita bread. Sprinkle with dairy-free cheese and add toppings. Bake at 400°F for 10-12 minutes until cheese is melted.

3. Snacks

Apple Sandwiches
Ingredients: 2 apples (cored and sliced), 1/4 cup sunflower seed butter, 1/4 cup raisins
Instructions: Spread sunflower seed butter on apple slices. Sprinkle with raisins and top with another apple slice to make a sandwich.

Veggie Sticks with Hummus
Ingredients: Assorted vegetable sticks (carrots, cucumbers, bell peppers), 1 cup homemade hummus
Instructions: Arrange vegetable sticks on a plate and serve with a bowl of hummus for dipping.

4. Desserts
Chocolate Avocado Pudding
Ingredients: 2 ripe avocados, 1/4 cup cocoa powder, 1/4 cup honey, 1 teaspoon vanilla extract
Instructions: Blend all ingredients until smooth. chill for a while before serving.

Frozen Banana Pops

Ingredients: 4 bananas (halved), 1/2 cup dark chocolate chips (melted), 1/4 cup crushed nuts or seeds (optional)

Instructions: Insert a popsicle stick into each banana half. Dip in melted chocolate and roll in crushed nuts or seeds if desired. Freeze until chocolate is set.

Tips for Picky Eaters

Managing picky eaters can be challenging, especially with food allergies.

tips to encourage healthy eating habits:

Get Creative: Present food in fun shapes or colorful arrangements to make meals more appealing.

Involve Kids: Let children help with meal preparation to increase their interest in trying new foods.

Offer Choices: Provide a variety of allergy-friendly options and let kids choose what they want to eat.

Be Patient: Introduce new foods gradually and be patient with their preferences and tastes.

Allergy-Friendly Lunchbox Ideas
Packing allergy-friendly lunchboxes ensures kids have safe and nutritious meals at school or on the go. Here are some ideas:

Wraps and Sandwiches: Gluten-free wraps with turkey and avocado, or sunflower seed butter and jelly sandwiches on gluten-free bread.

Bento Boxes: Include a variety of small portions like veggie sticks, hummus, fruit slices, and gluten-free crackers.

Leftovers: Pack leftovers from dinner, such as chicken veggie nuggets or mini pita pizzas, in a thermos to keep them warm.

Chapter 6 aims to make mealtime enjoyable and stress-free for children with food allergies. By offering fun recipes, tips for managing picky eaters, and lunchbox ideas, parents can ensure their kids receive nutritious and safe meals that cater to their dietary needs.

CHAPTER 7

EMOTIONAL AND SOCIAL ASPECTS OF LIVING WITH FOOD ALLERGIES

Living with food allergies involves more than just dietary adjustments; it also impacts emotional well-being and social interactions. Chapter 7 of "Deliciously Allergy-Friendly: A Cookbook for Healthy Living" addresses the emotional and social challenges faced by individuals with food allergies and offers strategies for managing these aspects effectively.

Emotional Impact of Food Allergies

1. Anxiety and Stress
Constant Vigilance: The need to constantly monitor food choices can lead to heightened anxiety and stress.

Fear of Reactions: The possibility of an allergic reaction can cause fear and impact overall mental health.

Strategies for Managing Anxiety and Stress

Education: Knowledge about food allergies and emergency procedures can empower individuals and reduce anxiety.

Therapy and Support Groups: Professional counseling and support groups provide a platform to share experiences and receive emotional support.

2. Feeling Different or Isolated

Social Isolation: Avoiding social events due to food allergy concerns can lead to feelings of loneliness and isolation.

Self-Consciousness: Being different from peers can affect self-esteem, especially in children and teenagers.

Strategies for Overcoming Isolation

Open Communication: Talk openly with friends and family about your food allergies to foster understanding and support.

Social Networks: Join online communities or local groups for individuals with food allergies to connect with others facing similar challenges.

Inclusive Activities: Suggest non-food-related activities or events to friends and family to reduce the focus on food.

Social Challenges and Solutions

1. *Attending Social Events*

Feeling Left Out: Social gatherings often center around food, making it difficult for those with food allergies to fully participate.

Managing Food Safely: Ensuring food safety in a social setting can be challenging.

Strategies for Social Events

Host Events: By hosting, you can control the menu and ensure all dishes are safe for you.

Bring Your Own Food: Bringing your own allergen-free dish ensures you have something safe to eat and can share with others.

Communicate with Hosts: Inform hosts about your allergies in advance and discuss the menu to identify safe options.

2. School and Workplace Considerations

Children in School: Managing food allergies in a school setting requires coordination with teachers and school staff.

Adults at Work: Navigating office lunches, potlucks, and meetings with food can be challenging.

Strategies for Schools and Workplaces

Create an Action Plan: Work with school staff or employers to develop an allergy action plan that includes emergency procedures and safe food policies.

Educate Peers and Colleagues: Provide information about food allergies to classmates or coworkers to foster a supportive environment.

Safe Snacks and Meals: Keep a stash of safe snacks or meals at school or work to ensure you always have something to eat.

Building a Supportive Environment

1. Family and Friends
Educating Loved Ones: Ensure family and friends understand your food allergies and how to support you.
Involving Others: Encourage loved ones to learn about safe cooking practices and participate in preparing allergy-friendly meals.
2. Medical and Professional Support
Regular Check-Ups: Schedule regular visits with an allergist to monitor and manage your food allergies effectively.
Counseling Services: Seek professional counseling to address emotional challenges and develop coping strategies.

3. Advocacy and Awareness

Advocate for Yourself: Speak up about your needs and educate others about food allergies.

Raise Awareness: Participate in awareness campaigns or advocacy groups to promote better understanding and support for individuals with food allergies.

CHAPTER 8

RESOURCES

Living with food allergies requires continuous education, support, and access to reliable resources. This section provides a comprehensive list of valuable resources to help you manage your food allergies effectively, stay informed about the latest research, and connect with supportive communities.

Online Resources and Websites

Food Allergy Research & Education (FARE)
Website: foodallergy.org
FARE is a leading organization dedicated to improving the quality of life and health of individuals with food allergies. Their website

offers a wealth of information on food allergies, including educational resources, research updates, and advocacy initiatives.

Allergy & Asthma Network

Website: allergyasthmanetwork.org
This nonprofit organization focuses on improving the lives of those with allergies, asthma, and related conditions. They provide resources on managing allergies, patient education, and advocacy.

AllergyEats

Website: allergyeats.com
AllergyEats is a guide to allergy-friendly restaurants across the United States. Users can search for restaurants, read reviews, and find detailed information on how different establishments accommodate food allergies.

Support Groups and Communities

Food Allergy Support Groups

Many local communities have support groups for individuals and families managing food allergies. These groups provide a platform to share experiences, exchange tips, and offer emotional support.

Online Forums and Social Media Groups
Platforms like Facebook, Reddit, and specialized forums host numerous groups dedicated to food allergy support. These online communities allow you to connect with others, ask questions, and share advice.

FARE Support Groups
FARE offers a directory of local support groups across the United States, providing opportunities to connect with others facing similar challenges.

Educational and Emergency Resources

Epinephrine Auto-Injectors
Familiarize yourself with the proper use of epinephrine auto-injectors, such as EpiPen, Auvi-Q, or generic versions. Ensure you and those around you know how to use them in case of an allergic reaction.

Medical Identification Jewelry
Wearing medical ID bracelets or necklaces can provide crucial information to first responders in an emergency, ensuring prompt and appropriate treatment.
Emergency Action Plans

Work with your allergist to develop a personalized emergency action plan detailing how to recognize and respond to allergic reactions. Share this plan with caregivers, teachers, and close contacts.

Organizations like FARE, AAAAI, and local allergy networks often host workshops and webinars on managing food allergies, providing valuable education and resources.
By utilizing these resources, you can stay informed, find support, and effectively manage your food allergies. Remember, managing food allergies is a continuous journey, and having access to reliable information and a supportive community can

make all the difference in living a safe, healthy, and fulfilling life.

Conclusion

Living with food allergies can be challenging, but with the right knowledge, strategies, and support, it is entirely possible to lead a healthy, fulfilling, and deliciously satisfying life. "Deliciously Allergy-Friendly: A Cookbook for Healthy Living" is designed to be your comprehensive guide and companion on this journey.

Throughout this book, we've explored various aspects of managing food allergies, from understanding the science behind allergic reactions to creating a safe kitchen environment, meal planning, and navigating social situations. We've provided a diverse array of recipes that cater to common food allergies, ensuring you can enjoy a wide variety of meals without compromising on taste or nutrition.

In the Introduction, we set the stage for understanding the prevalence and impact of food allergies, emphasizing the importance of informed and careful management. We delved into the intricacies of Understanding

Food Allergies in Chapter 1, providing a solid foundation for recognizing and diagnosing food allergies.

Chapter 2, Setting Up an Allergy-Friendly Kitchen, offered practical tips for creating a safe cooking space, while Chapter 3, Allergy-Friendly Ingredients and Substitutions, empowered you with knowledge on alternative ingredients that can seamlessly replace common allergens in your favorite recipes.

Chapter 4, Recipes, served as the heart of this book, featuring a wide range of delicious, allergy-friendly meals for every occasion. From breakfast to desserts, we've ensured that you have a variety of options to keep your meals exciting and satisfying.

Chapter 5, Meal Planning and Prep, and Chapter 6, special occasions and holidays, equipped you with essential skills for efficient meal planning, safe grocery shopping, and understanding food labels to avoid hidden allergens.

In Chapter 7, Kids' Corner, we focused on making mealtime enjoyable for children with food allergies, offering fun recipes and practical tips for parents. Chapter 8, Emotional and Social Aspects of Living with Food Allergies, and Chapter 9, addressed the broader challenges of managing food allergies in daily life, providing strategies for dining out, traveling, and handling social situations.

The journey of living with food allergies is ongoing, and it's important to stay informed, proactive, and connected with a supportive community. Remember you are not alone in this . There are many resources, communities, and professionals available to support you.

We hope this cookbook has inspired you to explore new culinary horizons and has provided you with the tools and confidence to manage your food allergies effectively. May your kitchen be a place of safety, creativity, and joy, where you can create delicious meals that nourish your body and soul.

Thank you for going through this journey with us. Here's to a deliciously allergy-friendly life!